How N

When You

By Steve MacGregor

First Printing 2015

ISBN: 978-1fifty8762164

Disclaimer

Dedication

To Julie. For helping me not to be fat.

Contents

Part 4: How not to be fat

Part 5: Final Thoughts

About the Author

Preface

Being fat is a problem at any age. It can make you unhappy, it will make you unfit and it may lead to health issues which can shorten your life or at least make your remaining years less enjoyable than they might otherwise be. Being fat when you're over fifty can seem like an even bigger problem. People over fifty often have very busy lives and may be at the most intense part of their careers. Putting on weight and getting unfit may seem inevitable, and doing something about the problem can feel like too much effort to fit into a hectic schedule. But it doesn't have to be that way.

Want to know a funny little secret about losing weight and staying fit when you're over fifty? Well here it is: There is no secret. Nor is there a pill, diet or food supplement which will allow you to get fit and lose that weight effortlessly, quickly and sustainably. Sorry about that. Not being fat when you're over fifty is the same as not being fat when you're younger, only more so. Eat the wrong stuff and get too little exercise and you'll get fat. Eat the right stuff and get more exercise and you'll lose weight. But to remain fit and keep that weight off, you need to establish a healthier balance of exercise and food which you can maintain not just for a week or a month, but for the rest of your life.

And that's what this book is about. It provides advice on how you can make sensible, sustainable and positive changes to your life. It also explains why being fat is more likely when you're over fifty and why that's not a good thing. You'll also find discussion of healthy and

1

unhealthy foods, but this isn't a diet book and you won't find detailed meal plans or eating advice.

This book is primarily intended for men over fifty who are overweight and unfit. And there are lots of those around. People are fatter and less healthy than they have ever been. Obesity and the health problems associated with it are reaching epidemic proportions amongst older men in the developed world.

Of course, being overweight and unfit are issues for people of both sexes and all ages, so why write a book just for older men? Mainly because I'm a man, I'm over fifty, I was fat and now I'm not. Which allows me some insight into the problems and the solutions. And because it seems to me that there are already large numbers of books and magazines providing advice and guidance for younger men and women of all ages. But relatively little for us older guys who want to lose weight and improve our fitness while maintaining a balanced and enjoyable life.

Introduction

So, you're over fifty and you're fat? The bad news is that you're causing yourself a number of long and short-term health problems as well as negatively impacting your self-esteem and your ability to do the things you want. The good news is, you're not alone - lots of men over fifty have the same problem. The big question is: What are you going to do about it? There are really just two options: Live with it or do something about it. If you are content to carry around that extra weight and wear increasingly baggy clothes, then you don't need to read any further. Good luck with that. Off you go.

Right, now that all the happy fat guys have left the room (and there are surprisingly few of them), let's talk about the rest of us. The fact that you have bought this book suggests that you aren't happy to be over fifty and fat. The fact that you aren't happy about it is a good start, but now you have to decide what you're going to do

If you want sympathy, empathy or just understanding, I suggest that you find a friendly shoulder to cry on. This book won't provide any of those things. Instead, it provides straight-talking, practical advice. It's about how you can take charge of your life and make choices which will change it in the ways that you want. It's about how not to be fat. If you're ready for that, we can work together.

I don't believe that following any of the advice in this book will be in any way harmful or hazardous to your health. Quite the opposite. However, if you have any underlying health issues, or if you're concerned about any aspect of losing weight or increasing your fitness, I strongly suggest that you seek advice from a qualified healthcare professional before you make any changes to your diet or exercise routine.

Why should you listen to me?

You may be wondering why I feel qualified to give advice about weight loss for men over fifty? After all, I'm not a doctor, a nutritionist or even a healthcare professional. However, I am in my mid-fifties, I was fat and now I'm not. I have spent a lot of time thinking about how that came about and why so much of the stuff I had read about weight loss was unhelpful, discouraging or simply didn't tell me the things I needed to know. Which led me to write this book.

When I wanted to find out about losing weight and getting fit, I found that most of the guidance that was available seemed to be aimed at younger people. And it was very noticeable that most of the books and magazines had pictures of young men with muscle where I had wobbly bits and slightly worrying titles like "*Four Weeks to Total Fitness!*". Even I wasn't naïve enough to think that four weeks would give me rippling abs and a toned body. What I wanted was something more realistic, intended for someone starting, well, a little further down the fitness scale.

At 52 years of age I was around 2½ stone overweight, I wore trousers with a 36" - 38" waist and I was unfit and unconfident. I'm now 55, I wear 30 - 32" waist jeans and I am in better physical shape than I was twenty years ago. What happened to me wasn't a miraculous diet or exercise plan or some metabolism-boosting pill but a change of lifestyle. I was lucky - I moved continents twice in those three years and that helped me to lose weight and get fit. It also gave me a chance to think about why I had been unfit and overweight in the first place and how my change of lifestyle led to these improvements. In this book I share my experiences and give suggestions on how you can achieve the same results without the requirement to travel the world.

This book provides no-nonsense guidance on how you can make sustainable changes to your life after the age of fifty which will make you fitter, thinner and happier. All the advice given here is proven to work, but it will take time and effort on your part. There are no instant cures or quick solutions. If you want miracle cures, try the Internet. If you are willing to take sensible, simple advice on long-term and sustainable changes which can make a huge difference to your life, you'll find it here. You probably won't end up looking like one of those guys on the front of fitness magazines, but you will be fitter, thinner and happier than you are now.

This book is mainly intended for men, and especially men who are over fifty. However, most of the guidance provided here is also relevant to younger men and to women.

I have tried to write simply and honestly about my experiences and what worked for me. I have also tried to talk straight. For example, I often use the word "*fat*" here to describe being overweight. I know that some folk find that distressing and try to find all sorts of euphemisms for being overweight. I don't think that's especially helpful, so please don't be offended if I call you fat.

You won't find any pictures here. If you are not sure what a fat person, an artichoke or a burger look like, try the Internet. You also won't find any detailed diet or meal advice here (though I will talk generally about which foods are beneficial and which aren't). The Internet is a great resource if you want ideas for healthy foods and meals. This book provides a philosophy to help you lose weight and get fit, not a diet plan.

OK, are you ready? Then let's get started by thinking about why it is that you're fat at the moment.

Part 1: Why I am I fat?

If you're reading this book, the chances are that you are over fifty years of age and unhappy about your weight and level of fitness. But before we start to think about how you can change that, it's worth taking some time to consider why you are currently unfit and overweight.

What is this fat stuff anyway?

"*Fat*" is word we use a lot, but what actually is fat? Fat is one of the basic components of the human body. There are two types of body fat: essential fat and storage fat. Essential fat (the clue's in the name) is vital for the healthy operation of your body. Essential fat is stored in small quantities in bone marrow, organs and muscles. In men, essential fat accounts for about 3% of your total weight. However, the stuff we're really interested in here is storage fat.

Many millions of storage fat cells are present under the skin (subcutaneous) and in certain specific areas inside your body. This includes fat which is used to protect and cushion your internal organs. Storage fat cells are mainly used to store excess energy. In simple terms, if you eat more than you need for your body to function each day, some of the extra is collected in storage fat cells. This is a great idea for a hunter-gatherer with an uncertain food supply. It means that it's possible to store energy when food is abundant and use that energy to survive when less food is available.

However, most of us now have access to a reliable supply of food and if we regularly store excess energy in storage fat cells, we eventually get overweight. Generally, having too much (or too little) storage fat is unhealthy.

Gaining and losing weight - it's a matter of simple arithmetic

Your body is an amazingly complex machine. Like most machines, it needs fuel in order to function. This fuel comes from the energy stored in the food you eat. "*Metabolism*" is the term we use to describe the process your body uses to extract energy from food. The amount of energy in food is usually measured in calories. A calorie is the energy required to raise the temperature of 1 gram of water 1 degree Celsius. Which sounds kind of odd when we're talking about food, but it's actually a sensible way to measure how much energy we are consuming. Your body needs a certain number of calories every day just to keep it functioning. If you eat more than that number of calories, your body will collect some of the excess in storage fat cells. Storage fat cells are very efficient at storing energy - one pound of storage fat can retain the equivalent of 3,500 calories, enough to keep your body going for around a day.

If you eat fewer calories than you use, your body will compensate by burning some of the stored fat. The greater the difference between what you use and what you consume, the greater the aggregation or burning of fat. To paraphrase Charles Dickens' Mr Micawber:

"Daily calorie intake 2,500, daily calorie expenditure 2,505, result happiness. Daily calorie intake 2,500, daily calorie expenditure 2,495, result misery."

So, whether you gain weight, lose weight or maintain your current weight really is just a matter of simple arithmetic. If you eat more calories than your body uses each day, your body will collect some of the excess calories in storage fat cells. If you eat less calories than you use, your body will burn some of the energy held in storage fat cells. It's a brutally simple equation. If you want to lose weight you must burn more calories than you consume. There are no alternatives, no options and no short-cuts.

You may hear discussion of people who have metabolisms that work at different speeds and a slow metabolism is sometimes blamed by people who are overweight. It's certainly true that some people seem to be better at extracting energy from their food. However, this doesn't affect the basic approach. Whether you have a fast or a slow metabolism, there are a certain number of calories you need each day to maintain your current weight. The specific number of calories which individuals need may vary, but for everyone it's true that if you consume more than this you gain weight and if you consume less, you lose weight.

In addition to how efficiently your body extracts energy from food, the number of calories you need every day to maintain your current body weight also depends on a number of other factors like how old you are, how tall you are, your ethnic background and how active you are. There are lots of places where you can find guidance on how many calories you need every day to maintain your current body weight. At the moment, I just want you to hold on to the idea that there is an ideal balance between the number of calories you eat and the number of calories you expend.

But, aren't there other things that can make you fat?

There are health conditions such as an underactive thyroid which can make you more prone to gaining weight. Other hormone imbalances, side-effects of some prescription medication and mental health problems such as depression can also have an effect on weight gain. If you believe that you may have a health condition which is contributing to making you fat, you should seek professional medical advice and help.

However, these things are actually fairly rare. For most of us, we're fat simply because we eat too much and don't exercise enough. Don't hide behind the idea that an underactive thyroid "*might*" be making you fat. If you have concerns, get them checked out by a healthcare professional. And remember that changing to healthier eating and losing weight can help improve many medical conditions including mental health problems.

Comfort eating

We all lead busy and stressful lives. Sometimes we feel worried or miserable or bored. These feelings are normal, but people deal with them in different ways. Some people smoke. Some people drink. But lots of us eat. This type of eating, which generally isn't connected with feeling hungry, is called comfort or emotional eating and it's common in both men and women. It often involves eating high-calorie, sweet or fatty foods and experts have estimated that up to 75% of overeating may be caused by emotional issues.

Obviously, comfort eating doesn't work. That is, it doesn't make you feel any less worried, bored or miserable. In fact, it usually makes you feel worse by providing a sugar induced high followed by a low and/or by making you feel guilty. When you're planning to switch to a healthy diet, comfort eating can be a problem. However, the good news is that most studies show that increasing exercise and fitness levels and losing weight help to maintain a positive outlook and increase self-esteem, which also decrease the triggers which may lead to comfort eating.

I wasn't fat when I was younger, so how come I'm fat now?

As you age, your body changes. Some of those changes are sensible in terms of extending life. We are designed to be hunter-gatherers not couch potatoes. In simple terms, you need less calories to maintain your body weight as you get older. This makes perfect sense in terms of survival. In a primitive society you simply don't have the energy or stamina to find as much food when you are older as you did when you were young, but fortunately this is balanced by your body needing less food. Good news if you need to hunt and forage for food. Bad news if your foraging is done in the fridge and most of your food is readily available and comes pre-packed and oven-ready.

Most studies show that men's' metabolism slows after we enter our thirties. The rate of slowing is difficult to accurately quantify, but generally seems to be in the region of 5% per decade after the age of thirty. So, by age fifty-five, you are going to need around 12% fewer calories than you needed when you were thirty. I don't believe that continually counting calories is particularly helpful or productive as a means of controlling your weight, but it is a good way of illustrating how your energy needs decline as you age.

To do this, we need to do a little arithmetic, but don't worry, you aren't going to need a calculator. In 2002 the US Institute of Medicine (also known as the IOM, a non-governmental body established under the Congressional Charter of the National Academy of Sciences) published an equation which specified how many calories the average person needs to maintain their current body weight - the Estimated Energy Requirement or EER. An important consideration is how active you are. The more active you are, the more calories you need to maintain your current weight. Three different daily activity levels are used in the IOM calculator:

> **Sedentary** - a person undertaking the basic physical activities of normal life such as gardening (without heavy digging or lifting), light household tasks, mowing the lawn with a power mower, loading and unloading the car,

walking from a car park to a nearby place of work or shops, etc.

Low Active - Same as sedentary plus between 30 and 60 minutes of moderate activity such as leisurely cycling, golf (not using a cart!), walking at 3 - 4 mph, gentle exercise (without using weights), swimming, etc.

Active - Same as sedentary plus over 60 minutes of moderate activity as described for Low Active.

Your EER also depends on your current weight and of course each person's metabolism is likely to work at a slightly different rate, but here are the daily calorie requirements based on the OMI calculator for a man weighing 140 pounds and 5' 11" tall:

Age	Sedentary	Low Active	Active
25	2560	2795	3095
35	2465	2700	3000
45	2370	2600	2900
55	2275	2510	2810
65	2180	2410	2710

Notice that your daily EER declines by around 100 calories per decade as you age. At age fifty-five you need around three hundred calories a day less than you did when you were twenty-five years old, assuming the same activity level. However, activity levels also tend to decrease with age, so you may actually need up to 800 calories less per day. That means you may need the equivalent of a burger with fries and a carbonated soft drink less each day just to maintain your weight!

The number of calories in the EER is a guide only - the precise number of calories required varies from person to person. But, if your eating levels stay the way they were when you were twenty-five, and your level of exercise declines, by the time you reach fifty-five you'll be overweight. This is probably the single most common cause of being overweight in men over fifty.

Is it inevitable that I'll gain weight as I get older?

No. It's true that your body changes as you age, making it easier to eat more than you need and to gain weight. But this is not inevitable. It's down to the choices you make in what you eat and how much or how little you exercise. One of the most important things I want to say here is: **It is your responsibility if you are fat** (health issues excepted). No-one else is to blame and no-one else can do anything about it. If you want to lose weight, you must accept responsibility for being overweight in the first place and take charge of your life by making better choices.

Kind of scary, isn't it? It's all down to you. In some ways that can seem a little daunting. We live in a society where we expect other people to do things for us, especially unpleasant or tedious things. But taking responsibility for yourself is also empowering. Just as no-one else can stop you eating too much, no-one can stop you if you decide to get thin. You won't be reliant on anything but your own will and desire to change.

The Short Version

You're fat because you eat more calories than you burn.

You need less calories as you get older so the problem gets worse.

The only way to lose weight is to eat less calories than you burn.

Part 2: Why should I care?

Being overweight isn't pleasant, but, does it really matter? There is a great deal of evidence that suggests that it matters a great deal. Not only does being fat affect your self-esteem, contribute to your lack of fitness and force you to wear baggy, old man clothes it can also make you susceptible to a number of long and short-term health problems.

Health issues

Being overweight is very bad for your health. A study by the Rand Corporation in 2002 compared being overweight with the effects of smoking, heavy drinking and living in poverty to see which had the most negative impact on health. The surprising finding was that being overweight is linked to the highest levels of chronic illness - higher than caused by living in poverty and much higher than those caused by smoking or heavy drinking. Think about that for a moment. Everyone knows that smoking and heavy drinking are bad for you. But being fat could actually be worse for your health than either!

Being overweight is specifically linked with a number of unpleasant diseases and conditions including Type 2 diabetes, high blood pressure, heart disease, strokes, osteoarthritis, liver disease, kidney disease and even cancer. No-one seems quite sure how being fat can cause cancer, but carrying extra weight is certainly linked to increased levels of several cancers. These are all nasty conditions which can shorten your life and make your remaining years considerably less pleasant than they might otherwise be. Losing weight won't guarantee that you avoid all of these, but it will notably reduce your chances.

Fat is a particular problem for men because we tend to accumulate excess fat on our bellies. This is an issue because belly fat isn't just a layer of subcutaneous fat, it also includes a deeper layer of visceral fat which surrounds internal organs. Belly fat is particularly associated with health problems such as Type 2 diabetes, heart disease, colorectal cancer and sleep apnea.

Self-esteem

So, there are lots of good, practical health reasons for losing weight and getting fit. But, let's be honest here. Avoiding these potentially debilitating conditions probably isn't the main reason most people want to lose weight. Thinking about something that may happen a few years down the line just isn't a compelling reason to change our busy and comfortable lives. Logically it should be, but most of us are too fully engaged with the day-to-day and the here-and-now to worry about something that might happen in the middle-distant future. For most men, the main reason they want lose weight is either to get fit so that they can undertake a specific activity or, most commonly, because they're fed up with looking and being treated like Homer Simpson.

In human society, how we look matters. It's fashionable to think of this as a modern development, but I suspect it has been around as long as there have been people. In terms of continuing the species, this probably makes good sense. A fit and healthy person is attractive to a potential mate probably because we're unconsciously evaluating their ability to pass on a positive genetic inheritance to future generations. Conversely, unhealthy people are less attractive for precisely the same reason.

Being overweight also affects how people interact with you. If you're overweight, people are more likely to view you as lazy, ineffective and lacking willpower. You don't believe me? Think about your friends. Compare how you think about those who are overweight and those who are not. See what I mean? I think at some level that we regard overweight people as ineffectual. After all, if they can't control their own eating, how can they be expected to effectively control anything else? Now, I'm not saying this is true. For the record, I don't think overweight people are less smart, dedicated or hard-working than anyone else. But I do think they're perceived differently. In terms of your career, that may be important. Is your boss going to trust you with that vital contract if you can't be trusted to keep yourself healthy? Would you?

> **Warning**: I am now going to talk about feelings. I know, that isn't something that us guys like to do. In fact, it's one of the things we're really bad at. But it's very important that you think clearly and honestly about how being fat makes you feel. It's OK, I'm not going to make you talk about it to anyone else, but it is essential that you're honest with yourself.

Until I was around twenty-five, I was skinny. Really skinny. At some point in my late twenties, I started to gain weight. Gradually, imperceptibly. Until by my mid-thirties, I was definitely carrying some extra pounds. By my late forties, this had got worse, to the point that I was seeking "*relaxed fit*" jeans and pants with stretchy waistbands. But inside my head, I was still that skinny twenty-five year old. Which made it very jarring when I caught a glimpse of my not skinny profile in the mirror or saw a photograph of myself ("*Who is that fat guy sitting on my new motorcycle?*"). In retrospect, this dissonance between my mental image of my skinny self and the plumper reality was a problem. I didn't like seeing myself in mirrors or in photographs or videos. Getting naked in front of my wife was something done carefully, and if possible, in the dark. Even though it happened so slowly that I didn't notice, I was becoming embarrassed at how I looked and that was starting to affect my life in lots of ways, especially manifesting as an overall lack of confidence. And worst of all, the weight gain seemed inexorable and inevitable. Something that I could no more control than I could stop my hair turning grey.

Any of this ringing a bell? How does being fat make you feel? The simple truth is that for most men, being fat makes them feel bad. "*Body fascism*" is something that you may have heard about, though the term is usually applied to the portrayal of women in the media (because, let's face it, women are better at talking about this sort of stuff than we are). But it's a very real issue for men too. Everywhere we're faced by images of slim, healthy and generally fit men. On television and in movies, overweight people are provided generally for comedic purposes or as negative characters. Can you think of a recent television programme, movie or book where a fat character also provides an effective, hard-working and an all-round positive role model? Neither can I. Being overweight has a negative impact on self-esteem. Low self-esteem has a negative impact on every aspect of your life. Losing weight and getting fit will help to improve your self-esteem.

Increasing your self-esteem (as well as improving your fitness and exercise levels) will also help you to avoid comfort eating. If you feel better about yourself, and especially if you feel more energetic, you are much less likely to need to use food as a source of emotional support.

Fatigue, aches and pains

Carrying extra weight places additional strain on your back and on your knees and hips, often causing pain and discomfort. In my younger days, I spent time racing motorcycles, which inevitably involved crashing. As a consequence, I had occasional trouble with my joints, especially one knee and one hip. These were most often a problem at night when pain would keep me awake though they would also ache if I walked or stood for extended periods. Since losing weight, I haven't suffered any pain in either joint. Zero. I had assumed that the pain in my joints was an inevitable consequence of getting older, but I can now see that it was at least partly caused by the additional weight I was carrying. It is claimed that losing just 5% of your body weight in six months can make an notable improvement to painful joints and contribute to avoiding osteoarthritis.

Being fat also makes you tired. Think for a moment about the extra weight you're carrying around. If you're 30 - 40lbs overweight (and that's fairly common for men over fifty), that's the equivalent of carrying a four year old child on your shoulders. For every minute of every day. Or a bag of golf clubs. Or the spare wheel and tyre from your car. No wonder you feel tired when you're overweight and that your joints and heart struggle. Just imagine if someone told you that you had to carry a set of golf clubs around with you, all day, every day, whatever you were doing. If you thought this was even possible, you'd object strongly. But that's what you're doing right now. Isn't it time you took that child off your shoulders, set down that golf bag and put that spare wheel back in the car?

Sex, fat and why your penis looks small

The low self-esteem that often accompanies being overweight has a major impact on your interest in sex. If you lack confidence and feel bad about yourself, you're not going to project a positive image for potential sexual partners. The fatigue that comes from carrying extra weight is also likely to reduce your interest in sex. Add this to the fact that men's libido diminishes over time and that men in their fifties are often at the most stressful stage of their careers (and that stress is a known sex drive killer) and it's no surprise that if you're over fifty and fat, your interest in sex declines sharply. But wait, it gets worse...

Being unfit and eating badly reduce your ability to achieve and maintain an erection. The link between fitness and sex is fairly obvious - the more efficiently your cardio-vascular system works, the easier it is to get and maintain an erection. The link between eating and sex is less clear but just as important. In men, insulin resistance which can result from eating foods containing lots of sugar drives down levels of testosterone in the body. Testosterone is partly responsible for sex drive, and after 40 years of age it tends to decline at a rate of about 1% per year in most men. Add a sugar induced reduction to this natural decline, and it's easy to see why eating unhealthily can lead to reduced interest in sex. But it gets even worse…

Fat cells produce oestrogen which negates testosterone in the body and tends to reduce sex drive. And finally, being overweight makes your penis look smaller. No, really! Even a perfectly respectable penis can look kind of unimpressive when it's struggling to peep out from under a large belly.

So, if you're overweight and over fifty, it's all bad news for your sex life. You're continually tired from carrying around that extra weight every day, you're embarrassed about how you look, your sugar intake is killing your sex drive, your fat cells are pumping out oestrogen to undercut your already dwindling supply of testosterone and if you do muster the enthusiasm to get undressed in front of your partner, your penis is going to look tiny. The good news (and I imagine that you're just about ready for some good news now) is that all this is reversible. Getting fitter, eating more healthily and losing weight will restore your sex drive and give you the confidence and physical ability to do something about it. And having a flatter stomach will make your penis look bigger.

Food and mood

The food that many of us regularly eat in the developed world contain things that cause our bodies not only to gain weight but also to perform badly. These include high levels of salt, sugar and saturated fats and a whole cocktail of chemicals designed to preserve, colour and even to enhance the flavour of our food. So why do we continue to choose foods that are going to make us feel lousy and get fat? Most men's answer is that the crap stuff just tastes so good. And it does - the companies selling this stuff aren't stupid. Most of us have become habituated to eating food that gives us an instant hit of salt, sugar and calories.

Think of it this way: you own an expensive car. Would you choose to fill that car up with second-rate fuel which will make it run badly and eventually destroy the engine? Unless there was absolutely no choice, I suspect that the answer is an emphatic "*No!*" And yet every day you do the same thing to your body. Food is the fuel your body burns. Fill it up with second-rate stuff that's full of sugar, salt, fat and chemicals and unsurprisingly it will perform poorly and will eventually stop working altogether.

In addition to affecting how your body functions, what you eat also makes an enormous difference to how you feel. I started to think about this after I had lived in South East Asia for over a year. The place where I lived wasn't a tourist area and there weren't any Western style fast-food places. So, I ate the same food as the locals, which meant lots of fresh vegetables, fish and fruit, very little meat and almost no pre-packed, pre-prepared food at all. Luckily the use of herbs and spices meant that even a plate of sautéed Morning Glory (a spinach-like vegetable found in Asia) tasted fantastic. However, just like every other person living far from home, I occasionally fantasised about a huge plate of sausages, bacon, eggs and beans. So, unsurprisingly, when I did return home for a short visit after almost a year, I couldn't wait to eat all the stuff I had been missing.

The result was surprising and almost instant. Within a couple of days of returning to eating high-calorie, fatty, salty foods, I was feeling sluggish, ill-tempered and bloated. My energy levels dropped dramatically and within a week, I was craving fresh vegetables and fish and the sight of a burger and fries actually made me feel slightly nauseated. I couldn't believe how quickly eating the same old stuff made me feel the same old way - depressed and tired. I had assumed that my improved energy levels came from my reduced weight and increased fitness, but I was surprised to find that they were also directly linked to what I was eating.

Now, I'm not suggesting that you need to go to South East Asia to eat healthily or even that Asian food is the way to go. But my change of continents forced me to confront the fact that what and how much I eat has a direct and immediate effect on my physical and mental well-being. If I eat crap, I feel crap. If I eat lots of crap, I feel really crap. I believe that the relationship between what we eat and how we feel really is that simple and that direct.

The link between what you eat and how you feel is fairly widely accepted by nutritionists and healthcare professionals, even though no-one seems to know why. The Mental Health Foundation has conducted studies that indicate that more than 60% of people who have good mental health eat fresh fruit and vegetables. There is a notable disparity between the reported mood of people who eat lots of processed, pre-packed foods and those who prepare meals from scratch. A bad diet doesn't cause bad mental health, but there does seem to be a link between eating healthily and feeling positive. My experience certainly confirms this. "*You are what you eat*" is one of those truisms which also happens to be true.

How fat is too fat?

OK, so it's clear that being fat is not good in lots of different ways. But how do you know if you're too fat? After all, everybody has some body fat. At what point does it become a problem?

In an average man in reasonable physical shape, anywhere from 10% - 18% of total bodyweight will be fat. So, it's unreasonable to expect that you will have no fat. The difficult thing is telling how much is too much. The most common way to measure whether you are overweight is to calculate your Body Mass Index (BMI). This is a simple calculation based on your height and weight which will tell you if you're within a normal, healthy range. Just Google "*BMI calculator*" if you want to give it a try. There are also a number of Body Fat Calculators to be found on-line which take into account other factors such as your age, sex and ethnic background. An even simpler way is to measure your waist - a waist measurement of more than 40 inches is generally considered an indication of an unhealthy level of belly fat.

All of these are useful if you want to be able to quote numbers to back up your concerns about your weight. But I'm going to propose a simpler measure of whether you are overweight. Does your weight make you self-conscious or unhappy or does your weight and/or lack of fitness cause you problems in living your daily life or in otherwise doing what you want to do? When you walk up stairs with a group of colleagues, do you notice that you're the only one puffing and wheezing when you get to the top? Have you stopped taking your kids (or grandkids) swimming because you no longer feel comfortable wearing just trunks in public? Are your walks with the dog getting shorter and shorter because you get more tired than you used to? Is your sex life suffering because you feel embarrassed about how you look or because you just don't have the energy or interest you used to? Have you turned down an invitation to try go-kart racing because you're worried that your butt may become wedged in the tiny seat? Would you just prefer to be thinner and fitter? If the answer to any of these is yes, maybe you need to think about losing some weight.

Now, the fact that <u>you</u> feel that you're too fat is kind of important, and very different to someone else telling you that you need to lose weight. I do want you to stop and think about this. My natural reaction if someone tells me to do something is to do the exact opposite. Not helpful, and it's a failing I recognise in myself. However, I know that many other men feel the same way, and for this reason simply being told that you need to lose weight is unlikely to produce results no matter how well-intentioned or sincere the advice may be. **You aren't doing this for anyone else: It's for you.** If it's going to work, <u>you</u> have to feel that you are too fat and you must commit to do something about it. That's a vital first step on the way to losing weight and getting healthy.

So, before you go any further, ask yourself two important questions:

> Do I feel too fat?

> Am I willing to invest some time and effort to losing weight and getting fitter?

If you can honestly answer "*Yes*" to both, great! It isn't complicated, won't cost any money and we'll discuss here how you can achieve it. Alternatively, if you're happy with the way you are, even if you recognise that you are carrying more weight than is ideal, that's fine too. You're probably not going to follow the advice in this book anyway, so maybe it's better to save us both some time and go do something more productive instead?

Are you ready?

Hopefully it's now obvious that losing weight is going to do all kinds of useful things for you. Your health is the single most important thing you have responsibility for and by losing weight and getting fitter you will reduce the risk of a number of long and short-term health problems. You'll also have more energy, your self-esteem will increase, you'll feel happier and your sex life will improve. These are all good things, but the problem is, you probably knew most of this already. But you're still fat. Why is that?

One significant issue is that getting fatter as you get older seems inevitable. If you look at your contemporaries, many of them will also be unfit and carrying extra weight. Why should you be different? This is important, so I want to spend a moment talking about it.

For most people who don't have underlying health issues or physical problems, becoming overweight and unfit when you pass the age of fifty is not inevitable. It's a result of choices you make. Your weight and physical fitness are a direct outcome of your lifestyle. You choose to be fat and unfit. If you don't like that, you can choose to change. Making that choice is probably the single most important thing you can do for your family and, most significantly, for yourself.

What's required is some fairly small changes to your lifestyle. Not a faddy diet or a short-term eating plan that you'll follow for a few weeks or months. These need to be changes that you can sustain for the rest of your life.

I'll explain more about the changes you need to make in the next part, but right about now you need to make a choice. Are you willing to accept that you'll spend the rest of your life fat and unfit? Or are you going to make some changes for the better? Remember, this is up to you. No-one else can do it for you and there are no quick fixes or miracle cures. You must want to make the change and be willing to make a sustained effort. You must own this. But no-one will benefit more than you.

Stop reading and put the book down for a moment. Think about the title of this Chapter: *Why should I care?* Well, do you care? And if you do, are you ready to make some changes? If you are, the next chapter explains what you need to do, but before we go there, you need to be sure.

The Short Version

Being fat causes many long and short-term health problems.

Being fat makes you tired and unhappy.

You choose to be fat. You can also choose not to be fat.

Part 3: What can I do about it?

If you have got this far, you'll understand why you are fat, why you are fat now when you weren't before, why it's a good idea not to be fat and hopefully you will have made a decision that you want to do something about being fat.

You're now probably wondering how you can achieve that, and that's what this part of the book is about. How to change your balance of food and exercise to ensure that you stop gaining weight and start losing it. No miracle cures, no quick fixes. Just common-sense advice on what you need to do.

You'll notice that there aren't detailed eating plans here. All of us like different foods and we all have different amounts of time to choose and prepare healthier meals. The actual foods you eat are up to you. What I want to do here is explain why some foods are helpful or unhelpful when you're planning a healthy eating regime.

More exercise, less calories

We saw in Part 1 that you burn a certain number of calories every day. If you eat less than that number of calories each day, you'll lose weight. If you eat more than that number of calories each day, you'll gain weight. There are two ways in which you can change this, which we'll look at separately.

- **Decrease the number of calories you eat.**
  Changing what and how much you eat will reduce your calorie intake.
- **Increase the number of calories you burn.**
  Increasing your levels of exercise will burn more calories.

Doing either of these things will change the ratio of calories eaten/calories burned. But the greatest benefit will come from doing both. Let's start by looking at how to reduce the number of calories you eat each day.

Food

Everything you eat or drink contains calories. Fortunately, most modern food packaging tells you how many calories any particular food contains. But calories aren't the only thing to consider if you want to change to a healthy diet. Some foods contain high levels of saturated and trans-fats, sugar and salt. None of these are good things. Other foods contain useful stuff like fibre, proteins, vitamins and minerals. Unfortunately, some foods contain all these things, good and bad, and it can difficult to tell what's actually helpful. In this part, I want to talk generally about how to plan a healthy, balanced diet while recognising which things you eat and drink may be making you fat and unhealthy.

The stuff you need to eat less of

Fat

We all need some fat in our diet. The problem is, too much fat can make you fat. And some types of fat are much worse for your health than others.

Trans-fats

You have probably heard of trans-fat, but you may not be aware of precisely what it is (I certainly wasn't before I started researching for this book). Although there are some naturally occurring trans-fats, most are created artificially, by adding hydrogen to vegetable oil to make it solid at room temperature. These are generally identified as "*partially hydrogenated oils*" on food labels.

You will find high levels of trans-fats in deep fried food served in restaurants and fast food outlets, in commercially produced baked foods such as doughnuts cookies, cakes and pizza and in some stick-type margarines and other spreads which are solid at room temperature.

Trans-fats are a relatively recent invention and it wasn't until the early 1990s that research began into their effects on health. However, there is now increasing evidence that trans-fats may be bad for you. They can raise cholesterol levels and can increase the risk of heart disease, heart problems and developing Type 2 diabetes. Eating lots of trans-fats will also make you fat. The health issues associated with trans-fats are considered so potentially serious that in some parts of the world

(Switzerland, Denmark and Canada, for example) laws have been enacted to limit or reduce the use of trans-fats for cooking. In the USA in 2013, the Food and Drug Administration (FDA) made a preliminary determination that partially hydrogenated oils are no longer Generally Recognized as Safe (GRAS) in human food.

Kind of scary, isn't it? So why do so many foods contain high levels of trans-fats if they're so bad for us? You can probably guess the answer - trans-fats are cheap. In addition, when they're used in commercial deep fryers, trans-fats can be re-used many times before they need to be changed, further reducing costs. Trans-fats also enhance the flavour of some food.

Trans-fats are something you're going to want to avoid as far as possible in a healthy, balanced diet. You can check food labelling to find out how much trans-fat is present in any packaged food, but in general you'll find trans-fats:

- **In most deep-fried fast foods,**
- **In commercially produced baked foods such as cookies, doughnuts and frozen pizza,**
- **In margarine and other spreads which are solid at room temperature.**

As part of a healthy diet, you should plan to reduce your intake of trans-fat.

Saturated fat

Saturated fats are naturally occurring fats which are typically solid at room temperature. You will find high levels of saturated fats in fatty beef, pork and lamb as well as in lard, butter, cheese and other full-fat dairy products.

Saturated fats aren't intrinsically bad for you, but eating too much food which contains high levels of saturated fat raises cholesterol levels and increases the risk of heart disease, heart problems and developing type 2 diabetes. Eating lots of saturated fats will also make you fat.

You can check food labelling to find out how much saturated fat is present in any packaged food, but in general you'll find high levels of saturated fat:

- **In fatty meats such as beef, pork and lamb,**
- **In chicken or turkey served in its skin,**
- **In lard,**
- **In many commercially produced baked and fried foods such as cookies, pizza and doughnuts,**
- **In full-fat dairy products such as cream, butter, cheese and milk.**

As part of a healthy diet, you should plan to reduce your intake of saturated fat.

Sugar

Sugar is a part of our everyday diet. It simply tastes good. There are two types of sugar in our food:

naturally occurring sugars (such as those found in fruit) and added sugar or syrup which is put in to food during preparation or at the table. There is no nutritional benefit to added sugar and there is good evidence that we are all eating too much of it. The maximum recommended daily intake of sugar is no more than the equivalent of six teaspoons per day. A recent study in the USA indicated that most Americans eat the equivalent of twenty-two teaspoons per day and most people in the developing world consume similar levels.

Why is that a bad thing? Well, sugar is calorie-dense. A little sugar provides lots of calories and increases fat levels in the blood. So, eating lots of sugar can make you fat, but it can also raise cholesterol levels and increase the risk of heart disease, heart problems and developing type 2 diabetes.

You can check food labelling to find out how much sugar there is in a product, but manufacturers are very good at hiding this. In addition to plain old "*sugar*", sugar can be identified in a number of ways including several names ending with "*ose*" (maltose and sucrose, for example), "*high fructose corn syrup*", "*molasses*", "*corn sweetener*" and "*fruit juice concentrates*". Some of these sound harmless or even healthy, but they all mean the same thing: "*sugar*".

Most people are aware that carbonated soft drinks are a major source of added sugar. One 350ml (12oz) can of typical carbonated soft drink contains the equivalent of ten teaspoons of sugar, almost double the daily recommended maximum. However, something you need to be aware of is that many fruit juices are not much better. Not only do these contain natural sugars, many packaged fruit juices have added sugar, even when they're labelled "*100% pure*" and "*not from concentrate*". A 350ml serving of apple juice for example, contains the equivalent of 9.8 teaspoons of sugar - that's only marginally less than a can of carbonated soft drink! And that's the high quality packaged fruit juices: some "*fruit juices*" are little more than fruit flavoured sugar water.

You can check food labelling to find out how much sugar is present in any packaged food (though this may be hidden using a variety of alternative names), but in general you'll find high levels of sugar:

- **In carbonated soft drinks,**
- **In fruit juices, especially commercially packed juices,**
- **In sweetened breakfast cereals,**
- **In chocolate, cakes and cookies,**
- **In some dairy products such as flavoured milk, yoghurts and ice cream.**

As part of a healthy diet, you should definitely plan to reduce your intake of sugar.

I also want to mention "*diet*" and "*sugar free*" carbonated soft drinks here. These probably sound like a healthy option - in these products, sugar is replaced with a cocktail of chemicals which reproduce the taste of sugar without the calories. Besides concerns about the long-term health effects of these chemicals and the fact that some of these products taste like anti-freeze, there's another issue here. When we eat or drink something sweet, our body produces insulin to help regulate blood sugar levels. It doesn't matter if what we eat or drink or eat contains real sugar or a chemical which mimics the flavour of sugar, the body produces insulin anyway. And what does your body do when it turns out that all that insulin in your blood isn't actually needed to regulate blood sugar levels? It stores it as fat! So, drinking sugar free or diet drinks can still make you fat.

Something you should also be aware of is that some products sold as "*low fat*" or "*0% fat*" (which may sound like a good part of a healthy diet) often have more added sugar than regular products. Removing fat affects taste (particularly in things like low fat yoghurt for example) and manufacturers often add more sugar to compensate. If you're choosing a low or no-fat product, do check how much sugar it contains.

Salt

Your body needs sodium to function properly. Salt provides high levels of sodium. However, just like sugar, we tend to eat far more salt than we need, and that isn't good. Too much salt won't make you fat, but it is associated with heart disease, increased blood pressure, strokes, kidney disease and congestive heart failure. So, when you're planning a healthy diet, you do need to think about salt. When you're over fifty, the recommended maximum daily intake of sodium is 1,500mg per day. Which sounds a lot. But a teaspoonful of table salt (which is made up of sodium and chloride) contains 2,325mg of sodium. Studies suggest that most of us are eating around 3,400mg of sodium per day, more than double the recommended maximum level.

Many packaged and prepared foods contain high levels of sodium, and not always the foods you might expect. For example, a four inch oat-bran bagel contains 600mg of sodium. A can of chicken noodle soup contains around 800mg of salt. So, even if you aren't sprinkling salt on your food, you're probably eating more sodium than is good for you.

Most food labelling tells you how much salt (sodium) is present in any packaged food, but in general you'll find high levels of salt:

- **In bacon, ham and sausages,**
- **In soy sauce,**
- **In smoked fish and meat,**
- **In potato and corn snacks,**
- **In gravy granules and stock cubes.**

Cutting down on salt isn't going to help you lose weight, but it is an important part of healthy eating. Try to choose foods that contain less salt and hold off on sprinkling it on your food.

Alcohol

Sorry guys, but we also need to mention alcohol. Beer is often seen as a particular problem, after all many overweight men are described as having a "*beer belly*". The truth is that for most men with a large belly, it's a generally unhealthy lifestyle rather than beer which is the cause of the problem.

However, you do need to be aware that all alcoholic drinks contain calories and all can help to make you fat (though some studies suggest that wine may be different). Just like everything you eat and drink, you need to be think about the calories you get from the alcohol you drink. The number of calories in alcoholic drinks varies greatly - a gin and diet tonic for example has around half the calories of a pint of beer and a quarter the calories of a pina colada.

So, if you remember the daily calorie guidelines in Part 1, one pint of beer can represent 10% of your calorie intake for the day. This doesn't mean that you shouldn't have a beer, just that you need to take alcohol into account when you're estimating your daily calorie intake.

In addition to providing calories and almost nothing else, alcohol can cause health problems if it's not consumed in moderation. We need to be clear what we mean when we talk about moderation.

Most guidance suggests that a man over fifty should consume no more than two 350ml (12oz) beers per day. And no, that doesn't mean that it's OK to abstain during the week and then have ten beers over a football game on Saturday. Drinking can also make you hungry and of course it lowers your inhibitions which may make you forget all about your healthy eating.

Now, I'm not suggesting that you need to give up alcohol in order to have a healthy diet, but you do need to think about how much, how often and what you're drinking.

The stuff you need to eat more of

Fibre

Fibre is an indigestible carbohydrate residue found in some foods. Fibre is good because it increases the intake of vitamins and minerals from your food and helps to remove toxins from your body. It also cuts blood sugar, lowers cholesterol, improves digestion by ensuring that food moves through your system properly and helps you to feel less hungry by making you satisfied for longer.

Most of us don't eat enough fibre. The recommended daily intake for men is 35 - 40 grams, but studies suggest that most men only eat around 15 grams of fibre per day.

All fruit and vegetables provide a good source of fibre, especially if you eat the skins. In addition, the following foods are high in fibre:

- **Beans, chickpeas and lentils,**
- **Wholemeal and wholegrain bread and pasta,**
- **Brown or wholegrain rice,**
- **Nuts,**
- **Bran-based breakfast cereals,**
- **Porridge.**

As part of a healthy diet, you should plan to increase the amount of fibre you eat.

Carbohydrates

Carbohydrates are an important part of any healthy diet. Carbohydrates do a number of helpful things including providing the body with glucose which is then converted to energy. Drastically reducing the level of carbohydrates in your diet isn't a good idea and studies have shown that a very low carbohydrate (ketogenic) diet can cause increased fatigue and actually reduce the desire to exercise.

However, there are many different types of carbohydrate. Some are helpful in terms of healthy eating and some are not. For example, fruit, vegetables and beans all contain carbohydrates. But so do cakes and carbonated soft drinks (sugar is also a type of carbohydrate). If you want to maintain a healthy diet, you need to be careful about the type of carbohydrates you eat.

The healthiest type of carbohydrates are found in fruits, vegetables and wholegrain products. These provide not just energy, but also vitamins, minerals, fibre and important nutrients. Some of the best sources of good carbohydrates include:

- **Fruit,**
- **Vegetables (but not potatoes),**
- **Wholegrain bread and rice,**
- **Brown pasta,**
- **Grains, seeds and nuts.**

As part of a healthy diet, you need to think about the type of carbohydrates that you eat.

Protein

Protein is also an essential part of a healthy diet. If you don't get enough protein you will suffer all sorts of nasty consequences like loss of muscle mass, decreased immunity and heart problems. However, the problem is not so much the amount of protein you eat as the type. Some foods which provide protein also contain other less helpful things. For example, a 6oz steak provides lots of protein, but it also contains high levels of saturated fat. A 6oz ham steak also provides lots of protein and less fat, but it contains 2,000mg of salt. A 6oz salmon steak provides plenty of protein, but much less fat and salt.

Some of the healthiest sources of good protein include:

- **Fish,**
- **Chicken (without the skin),**
- **Nuts,**
- **Beans.**

As part of a healthy diet, you need to think about the type of protein that you eat.

Minerals and vitamins

Your body needs a whole list of vitamins and minerals to function properly. The vitamins you need include B, C, D, E and K. The minerals you need include calcium, iron, iodine, folic acid, phosphorus and many, many more. Which all sounds very complicated. Fortunately, a balanced diet will provide all the vitamins and minerals you need.

Foods which naturally provide lots of vitamins and minerals include:

- **Leafy green vegetables,**
- **Nuts,**
- **Whole-wheat,**
- **Seafood.**

If you establish a pattern of healthy eating which includes lots of these things, you will provide your body with sufficient vitamins and minerals and it probably isn't necessary to take a vitamin or mineral supplement. However, if you do want to take a supplement, that's fine because your body will simply dump any excess vitamins or minerals.

Water

Drinking plenty of water is a good idea as part of a healthy diet, but there a number of misconceptions about what this actually achieves. It has been claimed for example that drinking water helps to flush fat out of your system (it doesn't) or that it will help you to feel full and eat less (it won't). It has even been suggested that drinking water helps to speed your metabolism and enables you to burn fat faster - there may actually be some truth in this, but the effect is so small as to be virtually undetectable.

So, why should you be drinking water? Well, your body needs liquid to function properly. Water maintains your body's electrolyte balance helps carry nutrients to cells. It's also an important component of blood and lymph fluid. Finally, a supply of liquid is needed to enable your kidneys to function properly and remove toxins from your body.

To provide your body with liquid, drinking water is a much better option than drinking carbonated soft drinks, fruit juices or beer. The good news is that it doesn't have to be bottled water. In most developed countries, tap water is perfectly safe to drink. Bottled water is just as healthy, but drinking tap water is cheaper and more convenient.

How much water should you drink? In part, that depends on your level of activity and the ambient heat and humidity where you live. Generally, your body needs about 2.5 litres of water per day to function normally. You get around 0.5 litres of liquid from your food, so you should plan to drink about an 2 litres of liquid per day. As much of this liquid as possible should be water.

Quantity

The other thing that living in Asia forced me to think about was the quantity I ate. Back home, I would regularly eat until I physically couldn't eat any more. You know, that "*Bleurgh!*" feeling, right? Over the next few hours the feeling of being too full would increase until I'd go to bed and spend the night bloated and tormented by indigestion. In retrospect, this was obviously a stupid way to behave, but for me it became the norm. I believe it's also normal for large numbers of men over fifty.

Part of the problem is the ways in which our bodies tell us to stop eating. Your body uses all kinds of signals to decide that it's had enough to eat. However, it can take 20 - 25 minutes for the body to analyse these signals and decide that it's full. I don't know about you, but I used to be able to eat a great deal of food in 20 - 25 minutes. So I'd continue eating until, suddenly, my body would say "*whoa!*" when it was actually well past the stage of being pleasantly full.

However, in the heat and humidity of an Asian rainy season, eating so much that I couldn't stand up unaided didn't seem such an enticing prospect. Suddenly I wanted to eat less, and within a short time, I became used to this. Now, I'm happy to eat much less than I did. In fact, I'm physically incapable of eating as much as I did in the past. I have also learned to eat more slowly and to stop eating before I feel absolutely stuffed, knowing that it takes time for my body to recognise that it's had enough.

As a result I almost never suffer from indigestion other than on those rare occasions when I return home and revert to my Western eating habits.

Eating too much is a habit. And it's one that you can quickly replace with the habit of eating less. Make a conscious effort to take smaller portions. Initially, eating less feels like you are cheating yourself, and you may find that you leave the table feeling less than full. But more rapidly than you will believe, you'll become used to it.

Superfoods, food supplements and steroids

There are things you can eat which provide lots of good stuff like fibre, protein, vitamins and minerals and not much of the bad stuff like fat, sugar and salt. Some of the best examples are fresh vegetables and fruit, nuts and fish. All these will help you to lose weight as part of a healthy diet. What don't exist are superfoods or supplements which will make you lose weight if you take them instead of a healthy diet.

However, you will see lots of advertisements for pills and supplements which are said to be "*fat-busting*" or "*fat-melting*" or which act as appetite suppressants. Most of these claim to work by making you less hungry or by increasing the rate at which your body burns stored fat. Sounds great, doesn't it? After all, if you can just take a pill to lose weight, you don't need to bother with all this healthy eating stuff. Unfortunately, there is one problem common to all these miracle fat-busting supplements and superfoods: **there is no good evidence that any of them actually work.**

Lots of people have spent time looking in to the effects of the various foods and supplements which are claimed to help with weight loss, and none have shown any notable or sustainable effects. Think about it - if there really was a pill which would make you thin, we'd all know about it. It would be headlines in the National press, not tucked away as an ad on the back of a niche magazine or as a "*click-here-for-amazing-facts*" link on an obscure web site. If something seems too good to be true, it probably isn't true.

There are also prescribed and freely available drugs which may help with weight loss. These have more concrete effects than the miracle food supplements - many work by limiting the amount of fat you absorb from the food you eat. However, even these drugs only work if they're taken as part of healthy diet. It's simply not possible to eat too much of the wrong stuff and lose weight just by taking a pill or supplement.

There are more natural things you can consume that are sometimes claimed to aid weight loss - green tea for example is often quoted as having "*fat-busting*" qualities. These things are sometimes sold as "*superfoods*" which will somehow restore your fitness while helping you to lose weight. Sadly, just like the miracle food supplements, detailed and exhaustive studies have shown that none of these actually work unless they're part of a healthy diet. And if you are eating a healthy diet, you don't particularly need these superfoods.

You may also be aware that some people use steroids in order to increase their muscle mass and to avoid fatigue during exercise. There are over 100 different types of artificially created hormones called androgens which are generically referred to as steroids. In the past, the use of steroids was fairly common and their supply was unregulated. However, the use of steroids can involve a number of unpleasant side-effects and in many parts of the world these are now available only on prescription and are used to treat specific illnesses and ailments. In general, I don't believe that you should consider using steroids unless these are prescribed for you by a healthcare professional. Steroids may be used by some athletes and sportsmen who push their bodies to extremes (though their use is illegal in many sports) but I don't believe that their use is necessary or desirable as part of a healthy lifestyle for most ordinary men.

Supplements, superfoods and steroids may seem appealing because they offer a quick fix. We live in an age of instant gratification. When we want something, we want it now. Being fit and thin is no different, so it's tempting to look for shortcuts which will speed things along. However, the truth is that improved fitness and sustainable weight loss take time to achieve. We're talking months or even years depending on how overweight and unfit you are when you start. Recognise and accept that now.

Now, most of these superfoods, drugs and miracle supplements won't do you any harm, other than making your wallet lighter. But they won't make you fit or thin either and there is a danger that they can distract you from what must be your main focus - eating more healthily and taking more exercise. So, my advice is to forget the pills and superfoods and concentrate on a healthy, balanced diet and a reasonable level of exercise. If you really feel that you need medication to help you lose weight or get fit, talk to a healthcare professional.

Food summary

Eating a healthy diet is actually pretty simple. Forget superfoods and miracle supplements, you just need to cut down on those foods which contain lots of fat (especially saturated and trans-fats), salt and sugar. You need replace these with foods which provide lots of fibre and those which provide healthy carbohydrates and protein. If you do this, you'll also ensure that you're getting all the vitamins and minerals you need. And if you can learn to eat a little less of everything, that will also help you to lose weight. Finally, drink plenty of water.

And that's it. Nothing complicated and, you probably knew most of this anyway. So, how come you're still eating and drinking stuff that makes you fat, unhappy and unfit? And how can you change? We'll talk about that in more detail in the next Part 4, but before that, let's take a look at exercise.

Exercise

Eating more healthily is one half of improving the ratio of calorie intake/calorie expenditure. The other half involves raising the number of calories you burn each day by increasing you levels of exercise. But exercise isn't just about burning calories. Research shows that a sedentary lifestyle is unhealthy for men over fifty. Regular exercise reduces the risk of a number of unpleasant conditions, including Alzheimer's, dementia, heart disease, diabetes, colon cancer and high blood pressure. It can also make you feel more positive and help you to sleep better.

The problem is, what type of exercise is best? There are all kinds of myths about exercising when you're over fifty. I have seen at least one respected web site which suggests that men over fifty shouldn't lift weights, for example. The truth is that any exercise is beneficial and you need to think about the type(s) of exercise that fit best with your lifestyle and which you can sustain long-term. Just like changes to your eating habits, you want to establish patterns of increased exercise that fit in to your life and which you can realistically sustain. A four week or three month exercise plan simply isn't going to achieve what you need. When you're thinking about increasing your levels of exercise, you need to think about things you can continue regardless of the weather, season or how busy you are.

Whatever type of exercise you decide to do, it's important that you don't rush it. Especially if you haven't exercised much lately. Trying to do too much, too soon can lead to pulled muscles, strained joints and extreme fatigue. Start gently and build up.

Gyms and health clubs

When we think about exercise, we often think first about gyms and fitness clubs. These are certainly a great way to improve your fitness levels and lose weight. However, the thing that no-one talks about is that going to a gym or fitness room when you're overweight can be embarrassing. Being around lots of fit, slim people just makes you feel more self-conscious about your man-boobs and wobbly belly. And some of the younger people I have met in gyms seem to view the presence of anyone over fifty as odd, possibly suspicious and maybe even dangerous (*"Is that fat guy on the treadmill with the red face actually going to survive? Do I know CPR? Should I call security?"*).

My advice is: hold off on the gym until you have lost some weight and got yourself a little fitter. If you do go to a gym, ask for advice from staff on the type and intensity of activities you should attempt. Start gently and build up.

Fortunately, there are lots of helpful exercises you can do that don't involve going to a gym and will still help to burn extra calories.

Walking

Walking is great exercise. Even better, it's free and you can do it just about anywhere. However, there is a great deal of difference between taking the occasional leisurely stroll and walking briskly and regularly. A leisurely stroll is fine for keeping your blood circulating and muscles functioning. However, the most benefit comes if you can increase your walking speed until you raise your heart rate a little. Ideally, you want to sustain this for at least thirty minutes.

However, if you're overweight and unfit, a brisk 30 minute walk probably sounds like a lot of effort. Especially when you consider that you'll probably want to be doing this every day. But, like all forms of exercise, start slowly. If you find that initially you can only walk briskly for ten minutes, that's fine. Keep doing this and surprisingly quickly, you'll increase the length of time for which you can walk.

A walk in the countryside is wonderful, but in terms of exercise, where you walk doesn't matter. So, why not try parking your car a little further from the office and walking the rest of the way? Or getting off the bus a stop earlier and walking? Or walking to the shop instead of taking the car? Remember the calorie chart back in

Part 1? What you're aiming to do is to increase your activity level to the Low Active or Active levels on the IOM scale. To reach the Low Active level, you need to do at least 30 minutes of brisk walking per day. To reach the Active level, you need to do at least 60 minutes per day. But of course, you don't need to do all this walking in one go. Adding an extra 15 minutes of walking on your way to and from work will provide the required 30 minutes.

If you really want to increase your levels of walking, think about getting a dog. Walking a dog twice a day will give you the exercise you need and a dog isn't going to listen to your excuses about why you're just too busy to take him for a walk this evening. Also think about listening to music or podcasts while you walk. This can help to make the time pass and you can use it to measure the length of time you have spent walking *("Yesterday I walked for nine tracks, today I'm going to do ten!")*. Also consider listening to the music you enjoyed when you were young. This is not only fun, it can help fool your body into thinking it's eighteen again, and full of energy.

For me, regular walking was an important part of how I lost weight and regained my fitness. When I moved to Asia, for the first time since I was twenty, I didn't own a car or motorcycle. I walked pretty much everywhere, simply because often the only alternative was hot, overcrowded public transport. I didn't set out to get fit, walking just became a part of my everyday activities. However, combining this with a better diet meant that within six months, I was noticeably thinner and much fitter.

I then moved again and had access to a small fitness room with exercise machines and free weights. At that point I was able to increase my levels of exercise while continuing to do lots of walking. Within another six months, I was in pretty good shape. Even after moving back to Europe and being exposed to the many temptations of Italian food, I haven't put on back any of the weight I lost in Asia. In part I'm certain that this is because I still don't own a car or motorcycle and I walk every day.

Overall, I highly recommend walking as part of your daily exercise. It's easy to do just about anywhere, everybody can do it and it is easy to fit regular walking into your daily routine. Walking is also unlikely to cause any of the muscle or joint problems which you may experience if you start undertaking more demanding exercise. Just keep it brisk and for at least thirty minutes every day and you'll be amazed how quickly walking will help your fitness to improve.

Other types of exercise

Of course, walking and attending a gym aren't the only way to get the exercise you need. Swimming, cycling and dancing are also good. As long as it raises your heart rate a little and you can sustain it for at least 30 minutes, almost any form of exercise is beneficial.

Jogging and running provide great exercise too. But these are things that you'll want to approach with a degree of caution. These are fairly intense forms of exercise which can place great strain on your heart, muscles and joints if you suddenly take them up when you're over fifty, especially if you're substantially overweight. Just like everything else, if you do plan to start running or jogging, take advice and start slowly.

Exercise summary

Increasing your level of activity in <u>any</u> way is good. Don't feel that because you can't run 5k or even walk briskly for 60 minutes that you have failed. Doing a little extra walking on your way to work, taking the dog a little further or spending time playing outdoors with your grandkids are all valid forms of exercise. As is anything which raises your heart-rate for at least 30 minutes a day. Start gently, and you'll find that you will naturally do more and more intense activities as you get fitter.

The Short Version

To lose weight, all you need to do is:

> Cut down on foods that are high in sugar and fat.
>
> Eat more foods that are high in fibre.
>
> Eat a little less.
>
> Exercise a little more.

Part 4: How not to be fat

By now you should understand why you're fat and unfit and the kinds of thing you need to do to change this. But before we go any further, there's something important we need to talk about:

Get your head in the right place first

Most men over fifty who are fat and unfit are that way because of choices they make. Of course there are people who are overweight because of underlying medical issues, but these are surprisingly few. We may not like to admit it, but most of us are fat and unfit because we choose to be that way.

Your health is the single most important thing you are responsible for. Getting yourself fit and losing weight will prolong and improve your life. And that is probably the best gift you could ever give to your family and those who care about you. But I want you to be selfish here. Only you can do this and no matter how much support and encouragement you get from others, putting in the effort will be down to you.

However, the benefits you gain will impact you more than anyone. You will enjoy and appreciate your life so much more if you lose weight and get fitter. No-one else can do this for you but no-one else will benefit as much as you do.

So, are you ready to choose to be thin and fit? Or are you going to choose to continue as you are? Please do stop and think about this for a moment. Changing your life, even in the relatively small ways required to improve your health can be difficult and challenging. In the early stages it can seem like you are putting in a great deal of effort for very little return. You'll be setting aside things that you probably use for comfort and emotional support, even if you don't realise you're doing that. It's not going to be easy, but the potential rewards are substantial.

Are you ready to make permanent changes to your life? Not just for a few weeks or months, but for good? If not, maybe you should put this book aside and return to it when you're ready. If you are ready, let's look at what you need to do.

The calorie ratio

Losing weight requires you increase the ratio of calories you burn compared to the calories you eat. As described earlier, there are two ways to shift this ratio in your favour. You could reasonably argue that both are blindingly obvious and based on nothing more than common sense. But for me it took a major change of lifestyle to truly recognise them, so I'm going to re-state them here:

- **What you eat and drink matter.** Changing how much and what you eat will have two effects, one immediate and one longer-term. First, eating healthier stuff will make you feel better right away. Your energy levels and mental outlook will improve and you'll feel less sluggish within a very short time. Second, over time you will stop gaining weight and you may lose weight. It's going to take time and it will be a gradual but sustainable loss, but it will happen.

- **Exercise is good.** Changing to a healthier diet will provide benefits even if you don't do anything else. However, if you combine a healthy diet with increased levels of exercise, the benefits will happen faster and will be more noticeable.

Everything we're going to discuss in this part is based on these two points.

Do I need to go on a diet?

In my opinion, no. Now, I know that this doesn't accord with the advice provided by many nutritionists, so perhaps I had better explain. For most people, a diet is a short-term change in eating habits intended to promote weight loss. The problem is, people view this as a temporary situation, and when the weight loss has been achieved they return to a "*normal*" lifestyle. Which were what led to them being fat in the first place and so, unsurprisingly, they once again start to gain weight. What I want you to recognise is that your current unhealthy eating and exercise habits aren't normal. They are a pattern of poor choices you have fallen into and which you need to permanently change if you're to lose weight and get fit.

When you start to think and plan for eating healthily, there is a danger that a burger, beer and soda-free life ahead may start to look like enduring a bleak and fun-free wasteland as you wait for your waistline to slowly diminish. Don't think of it like that. Eating healthily is not the same as going on a diet. Eating more healthily should involve a range of foods which you enjoy. You're not aiming to deprive yourself of good stuff for a week or a month in order to lose weight and then going back to your old habits. You are aiming to change to different foods which you can still enjoy, but which are healthier.

I'd also suggest that you don't weigh or measure yourself every day or even every week. Your weight fluctuates by small amounts for lots of reasons which are nothing to do with long-term weight loss. And after all, you don't <u>need</u> to weigh yourself that often. If you eat less calories than you burn, you <u>will</u> lose weight. It's a matter of simple arithmetic. By all means check your weight every month or so. If you're not losing weight, or not losing enough, you may need to adjust your calorie intake and exercise levels a little more. But remember, you're only aiming for a loss of about four pounds per month! If you're seeing substantially more than that, you may want to think about adjusting things the other way.

Most importantly, don't get obsessed with food, calories or weight loss. Obsession is something us guys find frighteningly easy to do. Whether it's striving for the perfect Star Wars memorabilia collection or knowing every last stat for the 2012 NASCAR season, we get fixated on things very easily. That can be good: after all, many jobs require a high degree of sustained focus. But it can also be bad. What you eat and how much you weigh are just parts of your life, they aren't all of it. Get things in proportion and make sure you still enjoy your life. And if that means going for a few beers occasionally or having a burger now and again, fine. That doesn't mean that you have failed or abandoned your new lifestyle. Within the context of a healthier life, the occasional indulgence won't hurt you at all.

Don't stop eating or skip meals

When you want to lose weight, it's tempting to drastically cut back on what you eat. After all, surely skipping breakfast (or other meals) is going to help you lose weight more quickly? Actually, skipping meals or drastically cutting back on your calorie intake is counter-productive if you're trying to lose weight.

Your metabolism works best and at its highest level while your body is digesting food. When your body doesn't have any food to digest, your metabolism goes into a kind of energy saving mode where it slows down the burning of calories. If you go more than four hours or so during the day without eating, your body will enter this energy saving mode. The longer the periods between eating, the longer your metabolism stays in this mode and the fewer calories you burn.

So, skipping breakfast won't help you to lose weight. If you skip lots of meals or cut back drastically on what you eat, your metabolism will stay permanently in energy saving mode and you may actually gain weight despite eating much less.

So, it's best to eat more sensibly rather than stopping eating or skipping meals. In particular a high-fibre, low fat, low sugar breakfast is much better than no breakfast at all.

Make a plan

Before you start anything new, it helps to have a plan. Fitting healthy eating and exercise into your life is no exception. You are going to be making some permanent changes to your lifestyle and if you're going to be able to sustain these, you do need to think them through first.

That doesn't mean that you have to produce a formal, written-down kind of plan. Though if you find it helpful to write things down, go right ahead.

What timescale should your plan cover? I'd suggest not less than six months and probably one year. I know, that sounds like a very long time, but think about how long it has taken you to get fat and unfit? For most people, these things take many years. It isn't sensible or reasonable to expect to undo years of bad choices in a few weeks or even a few months. A switch to healthier eating and more exercise will lead to weight loss and improvement in fitness, but these will be gradual. Most people agree that's the best way to achieve both these things, but it does mean that you are not going to see dramatic and immediate results.

When you're planning it may help to think of calories like money in a bank account. If you take out more than you put in, you'll end up with an overdraft. Put in more than you take out, and you'll end up with a healthy deposit. Except that in the calorie bank the deposit will be round your waist, and it isn't healthy. What you are

62

aiming for is to change the way that you eat and the amount of exercise you get to keep your calorie bank account permanently in the red by increasing your withdrawals (exercise) and reducing deposits (calories).

Having said that, I think that your plan should focus on larger changes to your life rather than micro-focussing on your day-to-day calorie consumption. Think about how you can eat more healthily in general and how you can increase your overall exercise levels rather than trying to draw up a minutely detailed eating and exercise plan. Considering every calorie may be appropriate if you're considering going on a diet for a few weeks. But, that's not what this is about. This is about making changes you can sustain.

If it's going to succeed, your plan needs to be five things:

- **Moderate**
- **Sustainable**
- **Realistic**
- **Balanced**
- **Just for you.**

Let's look at each of these in turn.

Moderate. Men aren't generally good at moderation. We're competitive and even sometimes obsessive. Why? I have no idea, but it does seem to be a man thing. Now, that can be good. It can provide focus and drive. But it can also be bad, because it makes us have unrealistic expectations which we are unable to achieve. When you're considering a change to a healthier lifestyle, drastic changes are not helpful.

When you're making a healthy eating and exercise plan, be moderate. Don't try to start too quickly or to achieve too much, too soon. If you suddenly switch to a high fibre diet, for example, you'll probably suffer from stomach cramps, pain, bloating and wind. If you drastically cut back on the amount you eat or start skipping meals, that won't help you get fit or lose weight. If your exercise plan begins with attempting a 15k run, you are almost certain to be disappointed.

In healthy eating and exercise, start gently and build.

Sustainable. As noted earlier, this isn't a diet plan, it's a change of lifestyle. The key is that you'll be sustaining this change. You need to consider how to make your plan sustainable. If you decide you are going to run 5k, twice a week, that will certainly help improve your fitness. But what happens when the weather is bad? Or you're on vacation? Can you still sustain your twice-weekly run? Perhaps it's better to incorporate two, 15 minute brisk walks as part of your journey to and from work? This won't improve your fitness as quickly as running, but there is probably a better chance that you'll be able to sustain it.

Healthy eating is the same. A radical change of diet isn't a good idea. Do the easy and obvious things first, and then gradually introduce other changes into your diet. By all means cut out that can of carbonated soft drink with your lunch and your visits to fast-food outlets three times a week, but don't eat foods that you find bland, boring or unappetizing just because they're healthy. Try new foods and flavours whenever you can. Try eating different vegetables cooked in different ways. Use herbs and spices to provide interesting flavours. We all enjoy eating and if your food becomes dull, it won't be long before you go back to eating the same old stuff. Do you like spicy chilli or curry? Don't give it up - try making these dishes with vegetables instead of meat and have brown rice rather than white on the side. Have chicken or fish instead of red meat. Swap those sausages in that casserole for kidney beans. Have a side order of green beans instead of fries or mash.

The ability to sustain the changes you make is essential. That's the difference between changing your life and going on a diet. A diet is short-term, so you only have to put up with things you don't like for a limited time. Changing your life means making choices that you can live with permanently. This may mean smaller changes than you would expect to make if you were going on a diet. Think about any change you are planning to make and ask yourself whether it's one you can sustain long-term? If not, maybe it's not the right change?

It may help to focus on short-term improvements. Healthier eating and increased exercise will make you feel better almost immediately. You'll have more energy, you'll feel happier and you'll probably sleep better. Losing weight is a long-term objective. It will happen, but so slowly it may not be apparent for some time.

Realistic. When you're making a plan to lose weight and get fit, it's tempting to imagine yourself looking like a young Greek god in three months time. Or running a marathon. It's OK, we all do that. But you also have to be realistic. It has probably taken you twenty or thirty years to get fat and unfit. It's going to take more than a few months to get back in shape.

If your expectations are unrealistic, you are going to be disappointed and there is a better chance that you'll give up. Be realistic in what you hope to achieve.

It's also tempting to set targets, especially for losing weight. *"I'm going to lose XX pounds in three months"*, for example. Again, I don't think that's necessarily helpful. If you set targets like this, you can feel like a failure if you don't achieve them which can tempt you to abandon the whole healthy eating/exercise thing. Conversely, if you achieve your weight loss targets it may be tempting to think that you have finished and that it's time to go back to your old lifestyle.

If you change to a healthier lifestyle, you <u>will</u> lose weight and get fit. How fast it happens or what your final weight is aren't really important.

Balanced. Balance is an important concept when you're thinking about making changes to your life.

A balanced diet is important. Your food needs to give your body all the protein, fibre, carbohydrates, vitamins and minerals it needs. If you were to eat just lettuce leaves and carrots, you'd probably lose weight. But you almost certainly wouldn't be healthy. Your diet needs to have variety and a range of different types of food.

But balance is important in other ways too. When you start eating more healthily, you're probably going to be cutting back on things that you enjoy. That Friday night burger and fries? The Saturday afternoon beers? The can of carbonated soft drink with lunch? Here too, you need to find balance. If you're overweight and unfit, you do need to change what you eat. But you still need to enjoy your life and have things to look forward to. Maybe you could go for a Friday burger once every two weeks instead of every week? Maybe you can have two beers on a Saturday afternoon instead of your usual six?

Remember, you have to able to sustain the changes you'll be making. To do this you need to be happy with your changed life. Being thin and fit is great, but if achieving this makes you miserable, you aren't going to be able to keep it up. Find a balance between what you'll be giving up and what you enjoy.

Just for you. You are unique. You are good and bad at some things and there are things you like and dislike. Your level of fitness, the amount of fat you are carrying and the speed at which your metabolism works are different to anyone else. The amount of time you have for exercise and for the buying and preparing of food are different. So, why would you expect that a plan intended for someone else would work for you? That's why this book doesn't contain diet or exercise plans. You need to do this for yourself.

Part of this means that you shouldn't try to compare your plan to what anyone else is doing. If you're currently taking very little exercise, then adding two, fifteen minute walks to your daily routine is an important and positive step forward. The guy down the street who runs 20k every weekend would probably find that pretty pathetic. But who cares? This is for you, not for him. Cutting out a couple of burgers a week probably wouldn't seem a big deal to that skinny Vegan couple your wife knows. But for you it's an important step towards healthy eating. Don't try to compete with anyone else, your plan must be just for you.

Planning for healthy eating

Let's start by talking about planning for healthy eating. We all have different lifestyles and we're all at different stages of unfitness and fat. So, as noted above I don't think it's possible for me to provide you with a "*one-size-fits-all*" diet plan. Instead I want you to think generally about how you are going to eat more healthily.

Look for the easy wins first. Do you drink a can of carbonated soft drink every day? Replace it with water. Do you regularly eat in fast food restaurants? Reduce the number of times you do this every month. Do you regularly eat to the point that you feel overfull? Then eat a little less. Do you eat a sugary breakfast cereal every morning? Replace it with a low sugar, high fibre cereal or fresh fruit instead.

Of course, these are the easy parts. The difficult part is how to modify the main part of your diet. If you're like most men, your eating patterns are probably largely based on habit. You eat the same things, most probably bought from the same place each week. You need to step back and look objectively at what you eat each week. What you're looking to do is to:

- **Reduce foods you eat that are high in saturated and trans-fats, salt and sugar,**

- **Increase foods you eat that are high in fibre and drink more water.**

The foods you are going to cut down on are those mentioned in part 3 and include:

- **Carbonated soft drinks,**
- **Fast food meals,**
- **Frozen pizza,**
- **Red meat,**
- **Sugared breakfast cereals,**
- **Anything else that is high in salt, sugar or fat.**

The foods you are going to increase are also mentioned in part 3 and include:

- **Fruit,**
- **Vegetables,**
- **Fish,**
- **Brown rice and pasta,**
- **Wholegrain bread,**
- **Nuts and seeds,**
- **Water.**

This isn't an exhaustive list of either the good or bad foods, it's just a reminder. What you're actually going to eat depends on what you enjoy and whether you have time to prepare your own foods. Your plan should look at your current eating habits and find ways to improve it.

Remember, you're aiming to find a new way of eating that ensures that your overall daily calorie consumption is around 500 calories less than the calories you burn. More than this may be unsustainable. A reduction of less than 500 calories per day initially is OK, it just means that it will take a little longer to lose weight.

Don't be tempted to skip meals (especially breakfast) to save a few calories and try not to go more than 3 - 4 hours without eating something.

Most of us already know what a healthy diet looks like, so planning for healthy eating shouldn't be challenging or complicated. What's difficult is finding food that's healthy but which you still enjoy and you'll be happy to eat long-term. There is no point in planning a super-healthy but dull diet. Unless you have the willpower of a Jedi Knight, you won't be able to keep it up beyond a few weeks. Focus your food planning on coming up with an eating plan that is healthier, but which you still enjoy. If that means initially that you just cut out some of the most unhealthy parts of your current diet, fine. Do that and build up when you feel ready and able. This isn't a plan for a few weeks or months, it's a plan for the rest of your life.

Planning for exercise

Your plan should also cover exercise. Think about how you are going to increase your daily level of exercise. Remember, all we're looking for initially is something that raises your heart-rate a little and can be sustained for 30 minutes or so each day.

Just as with healthy eating, you need to think realistically about how you can fit this additional exercise into your busy life. Going to a gym for 30 minutes every day is good, but can you do this every day? Is it better to start parking your car a little further from the office and walking the rest of the way? Or taking a 30 minute walk during your lunch break? Or walking each evening? If you want to track the amount of walking you're doing, get a pedometer. This will help you to sustain the amount of walking you're doing. If you can afford it and have the space, buying home exercise equipment can be a great way of getting exercise without drastically changing your life. If you enjoy watching television, try doing that while you're on your exercise bike rather than slumped in that armchair.

Also think about how you can change the level of exercise you get each day outside the 30 minute period. Are there journeys where you can stop taking the car and walk or cycle? Can you walk the dog a little further than usual? Can you use stairs rather than an elevator or escalator?

It doesn't really matter what form your exercise takes as long as you can sustain it. To ensure that you can sustain, planning is essential.

- Don't aim for too much exercise too quickly.
- Aim initially for around 30 minutes of exercise per day.
- If you can increase this over time, great. If not, just continue with 30 minutes per day.
- Be realistic - plan for exercise you can fit in to your life every day.

71

Just like your planning for healthy eating, your exercise planning must be achievable and sustainable. Initially, it's better to plan for a fairly low level of exercise which you can realistically sustain rather than attempting a higher level that you know you won't stay with for more than a few weeks. You do need to improve your level of exercise if you want to get fitter and lose weight, but it's often better to add more exercise once you have established a lower level as part of your daily routine than to try to do too much, too soon.

Think about calories. But not too much

We have already discussed that this is all about calories - Eat more than you burn each day and you'll gain weight. Eat less than you burn and you'll lose weight. But although your planning should take this into account, I don't want you to get too focussed on calories, and especially not on counting every calorie.

A sustainable weight loss is probably no more than one pound per week. To lose one pound in weight in a week, you need to eat about 500 calories less than you burn each day. How you achieve this doesn't matter as long as you keep that calorie bank in the red to the tune of around 3,500 calories per week. This doesn't need a dramatic change of lifestyle. Eating a little more sensibly and getting a little more exercise are enough to achieve this.

However, I don't think you should start counting the calories in everything you eat. Calories are a good way to illustrate the concept of what we consume versus what we use, and to explain why this leads to weight loss or gain. However, it's just too easy to become obsessed about anything including food, and I don't believe that's helpful. Instead, your plan should look at how you're going to switch to generally healthier eating.

Most dieticians agree that the number of calories you consume is less important than the type and quantity of food you eat and the amount of exercise you get. If you change to high fibre, low fat, low sugar foods, you will automatically reduce your calorie intake. Combine this with a little more exercise and you will lose weight and improve your fitness.

Don't get too focussed on how many calories you are eating every day. Instead, focus on choosing healthier foods.

How long will this take?

When you start out on a change of lifestyle intended to get you fit and lose weight, the temptation is to go for as much as possible in the shortest possible time. After all, you have decided to get fit and thin and you want it to happen right now! That's understandable, but it just isn't going to work like that. Dramatic diet change and weight loss isn't good for you and generally isn't sustainable. Studies show that most people who lose weight quickly put it back on again just as quickly. You're in this for the long haul. You're not going to be thin next week or even next month. But by this time next year, you'll be able to laugh at those fat pants with the stretchy waist.

Sustainable weight loss is probably no more than one pound per week. If you're 35 - 40 pounds overweight, it's going to take most of a year to lose that even if you're on-target every week. That probably seems like an awful long time ahead. But that's the kind of timescale you should be looking at in your plan.

It's just a habit

Most of our unhealthy eating patterns are a matter of habit, something we do without reasoning and sometimes without conscious thought. A few beers after work on Friday, a bowl of buttered popcorn while watching a football game or motorsport on television or a bar of chocolate during a movie. These patterns of behaviour are a problem. However, these can work in your favour because replacing existing bad habits with good ones happens fairly quickly. If you follow your plan and adopt your new, healthier lifestyle, you will be amazed at how quickly your new way of life becomes a habit. When this happens, it much easier to sustain the new approach.

This also applies to what we eat. Many of us have become accustomed to eating high fat foods which have lots of salt and/or sugar. When you initially eat something that is healthier, it may seem bland and lacking flavour. However, that will rapidly change. You may have to force yourself to eat healthy stuff initially, but more quickly than you think you'll become used to it and those high fat, high fat foods you used to enjoy will seem much less attractive.

How long will it take to form new patterns of eating and exercise? Psychologists have spent a fair amount of time looking at this and there have been a number of studies looking at how it takes to replace one habit with another. There isn't total agreement, but in terms of eating, around 60 days seems to be the norm to establish a new pattern. So, if you can sustain your new healthy eating for just two months, it will become a habit. Exercise too can become a habit though it looks as if this takes a little longer to establish. Studies suggest that forming a new pattern of regular exercise may take up to 90 days.

So, initially, you'll be fighting to change existing unhealthy patterns. But within three months your new habits will be working for you and healthy eating and exercise will have become something you do without thinking.

Persistence is the key

One of the problems with going on a diet is that this tends to be a short-term approach. You change what you eat for a time, perhaps you lose some weight and then you go back to the way you ate before. And most probably re-gain the weight you lost. The approach I'm describing in this book isn't about going on a diet. It's about making small but sustainable changes to your life. Changes that will become a habit and will become permanent.

However, that means two things: first you have to think in the medium to long-term - you probably won't see notable improvements in your weight and fitness for at least three months and it may take up to one year to lose most of that excess weight. Second, you're going to have to make yourself stick to this new regime at first. As noted above, after a surprisingly short time it will start to become habit and it'll get easier. But in the early stages it's going to be down to your willpower to keep going.

And you must keep going. It's especially tough at first. Your change of lifestyle will take effort and planning to achieve and you will see very little in the way of lost weight or improved fitness to sustain you. Be aware of this and take account of it in your plan. For the first two, or three or four weeks or however long it takes to establish your new behaviour as a habit, it's going to take willpower on your part.

Stay with it. It does get easier with time both because your new lifestyle becomes a habit and because you'll start to see improvements which will make it all seem worthwhile.

What changes can I expect to see?

OK, so you have made the change to healthier eating and more exercise. What changes can you expect to see and when will they happen? Of course, that depends on a number of factors including how unfit and fat you are when you start, how much exercise you are getting and how healthy your new eating habits are. Some changes are almost immediate. Some take longer to achieve. Here are some of the positive changes you can expect to see:

Reasons to be cheerful - eat good to feel good.
There are proven links between eating badly and feelings
of depression and low self-esteem. Subjecting your body
to sugar spikes, overeating and eating foods that are high
in fats and salts all contribute to making you feel bad.
Eating well, particularly eating a healthy breakfast
promotes calmness and positivity and provides you with
more energy. One of the first things you will notice if
you switch to healthier eating is that you will feel more
positive and more energetic almost immediately.

Confidence and self-esteem. Closely linked to the
above, switching to a healthier lifestyle provides an
immediate boost to your self-esteem. People with low
self-esteem tend to feel that they are out of control of
their lives. People with high self-esteem feel that they
are in control of their lives. Changing to a healthy
lifestyle can immediately make you feel more in control,
boosting your confidence and self-esteem. In the longer
term, as you lose weight and become more confident
about your body image, your self-esteem will improve
further.

Food, exercise and sleep. Millions of people suffer
from chronic, long-term sleep disorders and millions
more suffer occasional problems. This is a major
problem and poor diet and lack of exercise contribute to
sleeping problems. Studies have linked high calorie
consumption to poor sleep, and those who sleep best
generally have healthy, varied diets which include fruit,
vegetables and water. Being overweight also makes you
more prone to snoring and sleep apnea. Add to that
sleep issues caused by indigestion and discomfort from
overeating and it's no wonder that being overweight

interferes with your sleep. The good news is that eating more healthily, getting more exercise and losing weight will help to improve your sleep very quickly.

Sex. Generally, sex when you're unfit and overweight isn't great. Your confidence is low and your physical ability to achieve and maintain an erection are impaired. Switching to a healthier lifestyle will provide an immediate boost to your confidence, and as your fitness improves your physical ability to enjoy sex will also increase.

Losing weight. Now, you may wonder why this one is last on the list. After all, this book is about how not to be fat. The reason this is last on the list is because while most of the other changes you will see come fairly quickly, losing weight takes time. If you lose weight at a sensible and sustainable rate, noticeable weight loss will take time to achieve. If you're 35 - 40 pounds overweight, it will take a month or more to lose just 10% of this excess weight. It may take up to three months to see a noticeable physical improvement. Losing all or most of your excess weight may take up to one year. Losing weight is a long-term benefit. In the short-term, focus on the other benefits to maintain your commitment to your improved lifestyle.

How much weight should I aim to lose?

I don't think you should aim to lose weight. You should aim to eat more healthily and get more exercise. A natural consequence of doing this is losing weight. However, your weight loss should be gradual and may take anything up to one year to achieve. I also don't feel that it's helpful to aim to lose a certain amount of weight or to plan to achieve a certain target weight. If you do either of those things, there is a temptation to consider that you have finished when you reach your target, and that's not the aim here.

So, how will you know when you're thin enough? In just the same way that you knew you were too fat: If your weight no longer makes you self-conscious or unhappy and if your fitness allows you to do the things you want to do without restriction, you're probably in a good place. Because your weight loss will be gradual, when you do get to the point where you feel that you have lost enough weight, only a small adjustment to your calorie intake will be required to stabilise your weight.

Do I have to keep this up forever?

Being overweight and unfit is largely due to bad eating and exercise habits. If you go back to those habits, you will go back to being fat and unfit. However, if you can sustain your healthier eating and exercise regime for six months to one year, you will establish new habits which will help to sustain your healthier lifestyle.

Once you have experienced how much better healthy eating makes you feel and how much your life improves as you lose weight and get fitter, you simply aren't going to want to go back to your old habits. If you can keep this up for a year, you will have established new behaviours that should sustain you through the rest of your life.

The Short Version

Make a long-term plan to eat more healthily and exercise more. The plan must be:

- Moderate
- Sustainable
- Realistic
- Balanced
- Just for you

Your plan should be long-term. Six months minimum and preferably one year.

Part 5: Final thoughts

It takes time to realise that you're fat. And that you're not...

You may recall earlier that we spoke about dissonance, how what you think you look like and what you actually look like can be quite different. It takes time to get fat and you often don't notice this happening until something happens to abruptly remind you. Well, in my experience, it's just the same with losing weight. Unlike a short-term diet where you are thinking about losing weight all the time and looking for changes, if you simply change your lifestyle, you won't be continually thinking about losing weight. You will lose weight, but it will happen naturally and gradually and you'll quickly come to take it as normal. However a sustainable weight loss of around one pound per week means that it's going to take quite a while before you start looking like a movie star.

For me, it came as much of a shock to find that I was no longer fat as it had to find that I was fat in the first place. I had simply stopped thinking about weight loss and instead was enjoying the benefits of my healthier lifestyle. Again, a photograph caused me to re-think things. But this time the photograph showed a surprisingly thinner me, without a belly and extra chins. Suddenly, I realised I wasn't fat any more. Sure, I still had a few pounds to lose, but overall, I was actually in pretty good shape.

It was a good surprise, but a surprise nevertheless. I suspect that if you follow the advice in this book, you'll find the same thing. Make the change to a healthy lifestyle and enjoy all the benefits you'll get from that. And one morning you'll wake up to discover that you're not fat.

This is a time-trial, not a race

Whether you are planning healthier eating and exercise or actually doing them, it's natural to compare yourself with other people. But this isn't necessarily helpful. What anyone else is achieving (or failing to achieve) is actually completely irrelevant to your progress.

As we have said before: This is about you. It's about choices you make and the changes you want to make to your life. How soon or dramatically these changes happen just isn't important. So, don't be tempted to get competitive about healthy eating or exercise. If you do, there is a danger that you may judge yourself to have failed and be tempted to give up. Instead, focus on improvements in your life, no matter how small these may be. By sustaining small improvements you can make huge overall changes to your life.

Google is your friend. Most of the time

The Internet is a truly wonderful resource for information on just about everything. Losing weight and getting fit is no exception. The problem is you'll find everything from good advice by respected physicians to rants from people who are just a few short steps from being completely deranged and sales pitches for a number of dubious products. How can you tell what's helpful and what's not? In general, engage your bullshit detector! You should treat with extreme suspicion anything that sounds too good to be true and/or which claims to lead to an effortless or rapid weight loss or extreme fitness increase. To be sustainable and safe, both these things take time and any product or guidance which suggests otherwise should be treated with extreme caution. You should also avoid anything that suggests extreme or faddy diets which include a limited quantity or type of food. C'mon, you know that healthy eating involves regularly eating a balanced and varied selection of different food. Anything that suggests differently is probably unhelpful and may even be unhealthy.

You should also be cautious about any product which is being offered for purchase, especially diet supplements or other remedies which claim to help with weight loss or fitness increase. Anything that is described as "*fat busting*", "*fat burning*" or "*metabolism boosting*" is especially suspect. There is no reliable evidence that any of these supplements or herbal remedies actually work and some of them are very expensive indeed. Most of them don't do anything measurable at all though a few may actually be harmful. In general the adage "*If it looks too good to be true, it probably isn't true*" should be applied to anything sold over the Internet where regulations are considerably less lax than those applying to high street shops.

Where the Internet can be an invaluable resource is in helping you to find healthy eating recipes and/or food plans. When you are starting a healthy diet it's great to have a range of ideas on different foods and different

83

ways of cooking and serving and there is a whole range of information available on the Internet on both these things.

The Internet is a good source of information on the calorie, fat, sugar and salt content of most foods, including pre-packaged ready meals. In this way it can be helpful when you're planning how to eat more healthily.

The Internet is also a great way to find interesting and safe places to walk and run and gyms and fitness clubs in your area.

Short-term problems

Healthy eating should be just that - food that helps you to have more energy, better self-esteem and improved fitness. However, there is a possibility that the switch to healthy eating may cause short-term problems. You should be prepared for these, which may include:

Headaches. Headaches may result from a sudden reduction in sugar, salt, caffeine or even from a sudden lack of the chemicals found in many processed foods. You can avoid this by making a gradual change to healthy eating. If you make the change rapidly, I'm afraid there isn't a great deal you can do other than take pain-killers and wait for this to pass. Generally the headaches won't last for more than three or four days. If a headache persists for more than four days, it's possible that you may be allergic to something in your new diet. Wheat, rye, barley, corn, tomatoes, citrus fruits and some dairy products are all possibilities. Try experimenting by removing some of the new elements from your diet. If a headache persists for more than one week, you may need to seek professional medical advice.

Fatigue. A healthier approach to eating will provide increased energy levels. However, in the very short-term you may feel more tired as your body lacks the chemical and sugar stimulants which were part of your old diet. You may initially need to sleep more because of this. Within a week or so, this will pass and you will start to feel more energetic.

If you increase your exercise levels, this may also initially lead to increased fatigue. However, this will not last more than a week or so - increasing your level of exercise will also decrease fatigue overall.

Bowel gas, cramping and diarrhoea. Your digestive system and the bacteria in your gut take time to adapt to the digestion of different foods and a diet that includes more fibre. Any of these things are possible symptoms of your gut reacting to a change in eating habits. To minimise these effects, make the change gradual, introducing healthier, higher fibre foods over a month or so. Otherwise, be aware that you may suffer from these things but that they should pass within a couple of weeks.

Frequent urination. This is a normal effect of a new healthy eating diet. It is caused because things like vegetables having a higher water content than the foods you have been used to eating, drinking more water and because excess water will be expelled by your body due to your new diet containing less salt. Like most of the other symptoms of changing to a healthier diet, this should abate within a week or two.

Hunger. There will be times, especially early in your healthy eating when you will feel hungry. This is because you will be eating less and the foods you are consuming are more easily digested than some of the foods you have previously been used to. This will be most noticeable immediately after a meal, especially if you habitually eat until you feel stuffed.

You can offset hunger by eating more of the good stuff. If you are anything like I was, you probably do need to eat less too, but this is a change of lifestyle not a diet, so you don't need to cut back drastically on quantity as long as you're choosing healthy food. Lay off the fries but pile on those green beans! If hunger is a major problem in the early stages, think about eating healthy snacks (a piece of fresh or dried fruit or a handful of unsalted nuts or raisins) or chewing gum or even drinking lots of water. Happily, as your body adjusts to the new diet, you will stop feeling hungry.

Aches and pains. As you increase the amount of exercise you get, it's normal to initially feel some soreness in muscles that may not have been used for some time. This will pass within one to two weeks as your body gets used to your increased exercise levels. However, it's possible to exercise too intensely and too frequently. If you find that you have soreness in muscles or joints after the initial two weeks and which lasts for two or three days, you're probably overdoing things and you may need to cut back on the intensity and frequency of your exercise.

Don't give up

Having read all the negative effects which you may
initially experience by switching to healthier eating, you
may be wondering if it's really worth it? After all, if
you're going to end up bloated, headachy and with a
bladder the size of a basketball and you may not see
appreciable weight loss for months, why bother? The
answer of course is that, if you experience them at all,
these short-term problems will pass within two weeks or
less of your switching to a healthier lifestyle. After that
you'll start to experience the benefits that come from
your new choices, including increased energy, improved
self-esteem and the satisfaction that comes from
knowing that you really are in control of your life.

Don't let these potential short-term problems put you
off. Stay with it and the benefits will be more than
worth the effort. One year down the line you will be
thinner, fitter, happier and your chances of developing a
number of unpleasant chronic health conditions will be
significantly reduced. You'll also have more energy,
you'll be sleeping better, your sex drive will have
returned and you'll have the confidence and physical
capability to do something about it.

It's all about choices

For most of us, being fat isn't something that just
happens: it's a result of choices we make. Every time
you eat a high-calorie, high fat meal or drink a high sugar
carbonated soft drink or skip your daily exercise, you're
making a choice. You can decide that you want to stay
fat and unfit by continuing to make the same choices.

But if you want to take control of your life, lose weight and become more fit, you have to make different choices. No-one else can do this for you.

Even when you're over fifty, you don't have to be fat and unfit. It's your choice.

So, what are you going to choose?

About the author

Steve MacGregor is a Scot who was born in the 1950s. He spent most of his working life as a technical writer in the oil, gas and marine industries in the UK though he also spent time in Europe, North America and Asia. He is now a freelance writer for magazines and websites on topics including travel, current affairs, health and fitness.

He was thin, then he was fat and following an extended period of living in South East Asia he's now (quite) thin again. He is interested in stupidly overpowered motorcycles, large handguns, books and movies. He has two sensible, balanced, well-adjusted and grown-up children whom he occasionally manages to embarrass. He currently lives in the city of Bologna, Italy with his long-suffering wife Julie.

16535831R00053

Printed in Great Britain
by Amazon